Estrogen Dominance

Natural Remedies and Healthy Living

Table of Contents

Estrogen Dominance

Introduction

Congratulations and thank you for downloading Estrogen Dominance: Natural Remedies and Healthy Living. Estrogen dominance, like many other endocrine disorders, is a common issue which plagues many people the world over each year and can have potentially harmful or even deadly consequences. There are, however, many different steps that a sufferer can take in combating this disorder. In this book, we will go over some answers for some of the following questions: what is estrogen dominance? What are some of the best ways to combat the disease and heal from it naturally? What are the effects of high and low estrogen? Is this disease fatal? Are women the only sex to suffer from estrogen dominance? How do you cope with it? What do you do after you conquer it?

As you can see, we seem to have our work cut out for us. Not only will this book discuss some of the symptoms and causes of estrogen dominance, but it will also discuss some important information on other endocrine-related issues and how to maintain a healthy, balanced endocrine system.

The endocrine system is essentially just a large body of glands that release and produce the hormones which the body requires to function properly. One of the most important of these functions is the body's transforming calories into energy that will then power the functioning of the body's cells and organs. This function is disrupted by the deregulation of your endocrine system. The endocrine system also affects your heart rate, the growth of your tissues and bones, and even your fertility. There are also a number of other hormone-related diseases that are associated with the deregulation of your endocrine system. These include but are not limited to sexual dysfunctions, thyroid disease, growth disorders, and even diabetes.

All of the health problems mentioned in this book come back to the endocrine system, so this will be covered in depth.

There are numerous books on the market concerning this subject, so thank you again for choosing this one. Enjoy!

Chapter One: What Is Estrogen Dominance, How to Combat the Disease, and Heal from It Naturally

Estrogen dominance is a complex issue for a person to face. It is generally defined as the state in which the amount of estrogen is greater than that of progesterone in the body. This is typically caused by a decrease in a person's level of progesterone without a complementary decrease in his or her level of estrogen. There is, however, no set guideline on the amount of excess estrogen that constitutes estrogen dominance. It is determined by the amount of estrogen in relation to other sex hormones.

When there is an excess or lack of any given specific hormone throughout your body's endocrine system, overall imbalances start to occur and health problems start to rear their heads. Among other situations, this can occur when there is too much estrogen in a person's system and not enough progesterone to counteract it all. Estrogen dominance can be caused by a number of factors which only increase each year with the variety of consumer goods on the market. Some of these are listed below:

Excessive exposure to environmental xenoestrogens (industrial compounds often found in consumer goods like lotions and detergents); the use of synthetic estrogens such as hormone replacement therapy (HRT) and the birth control pills; anovulation (in other words, the ceasing of ovulation throughout the menstrual cycle, which is common in women above the age of 35); issues regarding digestion (which put strain on the liver's estrogen detoxification process); relentless stress (straining both the thyroid and adrenal glands);

incessant issues regarding emotional regulation; poor diet; and smoking, drinking, and adverse lifestyle factors.

As was mentioned before, estrogen dominance can have some detrimental impacts on a person's health. These include, but are not limited to: an increase in PMS symptoms, endometriosis, uterine fibroids, and fat gain on top of the abdomen and around the thighs, irritability, infertility, headaches, fibrocystic breasts, decreased libido, fatigue, and allergies. In addition, estrogen dominance can also cause menopausal symptoms, cervical dysplasia (a condition usually preceding cancer which causes unusual changes to the cervical tissues), as well as ovarian, uterine, and breast cancers (all of these are classified as being dependent on estrogen).

The various types of cancer resultant of estrogen dominance are obviously the most disconcerting elements of this disease. Cancer rates among the general population are increasing every year due to a wide variety of factors. The consumer goods previously mentioned that can cause estrogen dominance is an increasingly problematic source of estrogen-dependent cancers. One out of every three women is prone to developing some form of cancer within her lifetime, according to The American Cancer Society (ACS). In 1960, breast cancer rates sat around 1 in 20; today they are around 1 in 8. The ACS asserts that breast cancer rates have recently increased among women over the age of 50. Among the risks for this disease are long menstrual histories and the use of oral contraceptives, also progestin and estrogens for postmenopausal use. These risks sustain exposure to excess amounts of estrogen throughout life.

The link between excess levels of estrogen and various cancers remains an obvious one. Certain unhealthy estrogens can prove hard to detoxify as they are stored permanently in fat. There is also a link between obesity and breast cancer. Women who have higher body mass indexes (BMIs)-equating to higher body fat levels- also tend to have elevated levels of hormones, estradiol, in particular, one of the more potent estrogens within the endocrine system.

One of the best ways for women to reduce their risk of developing breast cancer is maintaining a normal weight. In doing these women can reduce the levels of potentially harmful hormones stored within their body fat.

Some important tips regarding protecting your tissue from excess levels of estrogen and restoring normal function to your endocrine system are mentioned below:

- Stick to a diet including organic whole foods and fiber and make sure to eat five to nine servings of vegetables and fruits each and every day.

Good sources of fiber, in this case, include brussel sprouts, turnips, peas, starchy vegetables (sweet potatoes, winter squash, plantains, taro), avocados, berries, coconut, beans and legumes, seeds (flax and sesame in particular), and nuts. A diet such as this one will ensure reproductive health as well as hormone balance.

- It is also important to eat foods which will support your liver.

Your liver is the greatest natural detoxifier that you have at your disposal, especially in dealing with estrogen. It does, however, tend to be fatigued though. One way to keep this organ healthy and functioning properly is to stick to a diet of herbs, dark leafy greens, and lots of filtered water. Herbs (such as garlic and cilantro) should be eaten preferably with every meal, 5-9 servings of dark leafy greens (such as dandelion, arugula, Swiss chard, and kale) should be eaten every day, and a general rule of thumb for how much water you drink a day in ounces is your body weight /2.

- Identify and decrease your amount of chronic stressors and take care of your thyroid and adrenal glands with lots of supplementation and rest.

High levels of stress throughout prolonged periods can lead to a decrease in progesterone production, which can, in turn, lead to symptoms of estrogen dominance. Cortisol is your body's natural stress hormone. This hormone is needed for the production of both estrogen and progesterone, which is why an excess of this hormone in the body can lead to deregulation of these other hormones. Prolonged stress, as well as the increased amount of cortisol that accompanies it, often leads to hormonal imbalances, as well as a number of other health problems.

Adrenal and thyroid glands are part of your body's limbic system. This system serves as your brain's fight or flight response headquarters. The persistence of cortisol within these regions of the brain is unhealthy and tends to build upon itself. This is where estrogen dominance can start to affect mental health, causing harmful and potentially dangerous side effects such as anxiety and depression.

What is unassailable is the fact that the modern world is filled with countless stressors, but how these are reacted to is entirely up to the individual's control. There are a number of ways to deal with excess stress. These would be restorative yoga, deep-breathing exercises, going on walks (preferably in natural settings), biofeedback, a massage, a hot bath, or whatever relaxes you personally. This is one of the most important steps in regulating your estrogen levels, as well as your overall health and well-being.

- Take probiotic supplements to restore any digestive imbalances you may have by crowding out the overgrowth of yeast and bad bacteria with good bacteria.

- Limit your exposure to xenoestrogens by using and wearing safe products void of things that may disrupt your hormonal balance such as phthalates and parabens. This may be the easiest and most effective way to limit your estrogen levels. Xenoestrogens are substances that are not natural and have negative hormonal effects on your body. Estrogen and progesterone levels behave like a seesaw in the body, when one goes up, the other goes down. This is why exposing yourself to artificial estrogens will decrease your progesterone levels, causing chemical imbalances. Xenoestrogens are toxic and unhealthy, being absorbed by the skin and gradually building up within the body over periods of time. Xenoestrogens, along with other xenohormones, can be found in the following products:

  o Farm-raised fish, non-organic meat produced from livestock that has been raised conventionally, car exhaust, plastics, products for body care that contain chemicals such as sulfates and parabens, non-organic vegetables and fruits (covered in herbicides, pesticides, and or fungicides), canned foods (containing BPA or bisphenol A), adhesives and solvents, PCBs from industrial waste, and emulsifiers found in soaps and cosmetics.

> Always be sure to check the ingredients of the products you buy for these and other harmful chemicals.

- Contact a practitioner who offers natural and safe relief for symptoms of transitioning hormone levels.

- Limit your use of HRT (hormone replacement therapy).

- Quit or limit alcohol and or nicotine use.

There are countless supplements that help with estrogen dominance and its symptoms. A few of them are listed below with their effects:

- Magnesium
  In addition to helping the body in absorbing calcium, magnesium also helps to regulate the pituitary gland, which then helps to regulate hormone levels. The production of FSH (follicle stimulating hormones) and LH (luteinizing hormones) is regulated by the pituitary gland, both of which then regulate estrogen and progesterone production. When your body does not have enough magnesium, it will then create less of the hormones necessary for keeping your reproductive system in working order. Keeping your magnesium at a healthy rate will help heal PCOS, PMS, menopausal symptoms, adrenal fatigue, and many other hormone-cycle related problems. Fortunately, it does not take long for these positive changes to happen after magnesium has been increased.

- Vitamin B6

This helps in the regulation of hormones. Taking B6 at a rate of 200-800 mg/day can help to reduce estrogen levels in the blood as well as improve PMS symptoms. Women with higher levels of B6 have also been shown to have improved their fertility by 120% and lowered their chances of miscarriage by 50%.

- Maca
  Maca is a supplement that can control the amounts of progesterone and estrogen in the body. When levels of these hormones are deregulated, it can prevent a woman from being able to conceive or decrease her chances of carrying the pregnancy to term. Maca is great for fertility because it increases a woman's chances of becoming pregnant in a healthy, natural way.

- DIM-Evail
  DIM is a compound which helps estrogen metabolize properly. It balances hormones by helping in breaking estrogen down and removing it from the body.

- Vitex
  This is one of the more powerful herbs on the market for women's menstrual health as well as fertility. Vitex is especially notable in its ability to regulate hormones while in itself containing no hormones, a trait that most supplements cannot boast.

Hormones play a massive role in your overall health. All of the hormones in the human body play specific roles in the health and functioning of the body. These, however, only work properly when they are set at their normal ratios in relation to one another. Hormones are in charge of many different things, including your weight gain or loss by regulating your metabolism. Hormones also control your digestive functioning, your energy levels, and the severity of mood swings that occur during periods. Hormone imbalances in men can cause erectile dysfunctions and low libido. They can even cause the growth of breasts in men, on rarer occasions.

Seeing as how all of your hormones work in relation to one another, it is not surprising that when one hormone is dominating, others deregulations can occur. This is where the undesirable symptoms mentioned above start to occur; as one hormone is typically doing too much of whatever it does while the others are not doing enough. In contrast, when your hormones are all in order and working properly, the rest of your body eagerly follows suit.

Commonly related to and often the cause of estrogen dominance and low progesterone is the hormonal imbalance typically caused by chronic stress, prolonged exposure to estrogen, and a diet lacking in essential vitamins and nutrients. It is advisable to consult your doctor to see what hormonal imbalances you may have and the best possible treatment options for these.

So, to recap, estrogen dominance is a disease in which estrogen levels rise to a point at which they become unhealthy, usually as a result of low progesterone levels. This can, in turn, cause a myriad of different symptoms, such as an increase in PMS symptoms, endometriosis, uterine fibroids, fat gain on top of the abdomen and around the thighs, irritability, infertility, headaches, fibrocystic breasts, decreased libido, fatigue, and allergies. The disease can even cause ovarian, uterine, and breast cancers as well.

There are, however, a few ways to combat this disease. These include maintaining a healthy weight, sticking to a healthy diet, taking supplements to support hormonal regularity, and limiting personal stressors. When all of these skills are practiced together quick progress can usually be made and health, as well as the quality of life of the sufferer, can be improved dramatically.

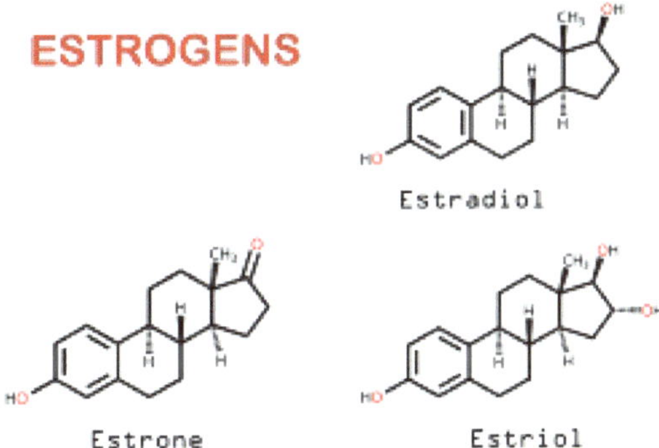

Chapter Two: High and Low Estrogen - What the Opposite Ends of the Spectrum Do to a Person and How to Balance the Two

High estrogen (or estrogen dominance) has now been grazed over, but an equally harmful condition is low estrogen. The hormone needs to remain at a normal amount for the body to function properly.

Low estrogen levels are often confused for menopause because of the symptoms that are pretty much the same. Menopause usually does not occur in women until around their 40s or 50s, and premature menopause usually hits women who suffer from it around their late thirties at the youngest, so younger women (adolescents to mid-thirties) who are exhibiting symptoms of menopause should look more into the possibility of them having low estrogen levels. For some, developing low estrogen levels is genetic. Others develop low estrogen levels as a result of ovarian cysts, thyroid disorders, or undergoing chemo or other radiation therapies. Another common cause of low estrogen is low body fat, especially around puberty, when hormonal changes are at their highest. There are a number of symptoms that occur with this irregularity. A few of them are shown below.

- Fewer/no periods
  This is actually the most common symptom of low estrogen levels. Estrogen is the most powerful driver of a woman's menstrual cycle. Low levels of this hormone can either make your period very light or make it go away altogether. Estrogen is the hormone which causes your uterine lining to thicken every month, which in

turn causes it to shed as well. Low levels of estrogen cause less thickening and therefore less tissue being released during menstruation, the opposite is true for high estrogen.

- Mood swings

Since estrogen is the main driver of your menstrual cycle, it would naturally follow that estrogen levels have profound effects on your mood. All of the mood swings that come with the menstrual cycle are all due to the hormones involved in the operation of the cycle. If estrogen levels are low, then the whole cycle gets off base, and mood swings can become more severe.

- Sleep problems/ fatigue

Estrogen production is closely related to serotonin production, a hormone which creates melatonin, the main sleep hormone. Having low estrogen is tantamount to having low serotonin, which in turn leads to sleep problems. Fatigue is a result of these problems.

- Depression

Serotonin also acts as a natural antidepressant, so low estrogen levels can affect your ability to fend off negative mental states such as depression.

- Low libido

Low estrogen levels can also curtail any sexuality or sexual expression. Serotonin levels also correspond to sex drive. The less serotonin you have, the less desire for sex you will typically feel.

- Painful Sex

Low estrogen levels can dry out the vaginal canal, making sex less enjoyable and even sometimes painful. It can also thin out your vaginal walls, leading to even more pain and discomfort.

- Dry eyes
  Estrogen can dry up more than just the vaginal canal. In addition, it is linked to the number of tears that your eyes can produce. Low estrogen levels can lead to your eyes feeling dry.

- Dry skin
  This is another thing that low estrogen levels can dry out. Estrogen is known to increase the number of natural acids in your skin responsible for retaining moisture. When estrogen levels are low, this can leave your skin uncomfortably dry.

- Hot flashes and night sweats
  These are among the symptoms that are similar to those of menopause. The hypothalamus is the part of the brain responsible for regulating body temperature. Low estrogen can impede its ability to do this. This can result in hot flashes and night sweats, both of which can further the progression of sleep problems.

- Troubles in remembering things
  In addition to regulating your levels of serotonin, estrogen also regulates your levels of cortisol as a stress hormone which helps neurotransmitters in the brain communicate effectively with one another. Memory lapses can occur when there is not enough estrogen regulating cortisol levels in the brain. The neural

networking just cannot work effectively without regulation.

- Difficulty in concentrating on tasks
This cortisol deregulation can also have adverse effects on your ability to focus. Coupling this with sleep problems leads to the near impossibility of focusing on most tasks.

- Increased headaches
Low levels of estrogen and turbulence in hormonal systems can also lead to headaches. Women typically get most of their monthly headaches right before their periods, the time at which estrogen levels are at their lowest. Combine this with already low levels of estrogen and migraines can start to occur.

- Having difficulties conceiving
If you are trying to get pregnant, it may be beneficial to check your levels of estrogen with a professional. As was mentioned in the first of these tips, low estrogen levels can impair the growth of your uterine wall. This can make pregnancy a challenge.

- Increase in weight
Again, estrogen connects itself to your fat cells. Interestingly enough, whether you have too much or too little estrogen in your system, body fat tends to increase. The only way to curtail this is by balancing out your hormonal levels.

- Urinary tract infections
One of the most harmful symptoms of low estrogen is the presence of UTIs (urinary tract infections). Low

estrogen thins out the lining of your urethra, making it easier for unwanted and potentially harmful bacteria to get in.

- Anxiety
  Low estrogen levels can also lead to anxiety. This is mostly due to the drop in serotonin levels. Anxiety in these cases is often made even worse by having to cope with all the other symptoms. You are more likely to feel fear when your serotonin levels drop to an unhealthy extent, and fear typically builds off of itself.

Abnormal levels of estrogen, whether they are too high or too low, are never healthy and should be dealt with as quickly as possible. The first thing to do if you are experiencing any of the symptoms listed above is to contact your doctor about them as soon as possible. It takes a professional to assess what the best treatment options would be for you in this case. Often this includes hormone replacement therapies for a brief period of time.

Low estrogen, or whatever type of hormonal imbalance you may suffer from, manifests itself within the endocrine system. Here we should take a look at what the endocrine system is and what exactly it does.

The endocrine system is a blanket term for all the areas in your body that produce and regulate hormones. One way to look at hormones is as being the messengers for cells and organs to communicate with one another effectively. Without the endocrine system, or at least when the system is not working properly, various parts of the body would continue to work independently from one another with no communication being practiced.

Some of the organs included in the endocrine system which produce hormones are the pineal gland (which sets our circadian rhythm), the thyroid (which sets the metabolism of cells throughout the body), the pancreas (which is involved in blood sugar control and digestion), the testes and ovaries (which produce the sex hormones testosterone, progesterone, and estrogen), and the adrenal glands (which produce cortisol to balance physiological and emotional stress in order to maintain homeostasis).

Throughout the day, the levels of hormones in the endocrine system fluctuate. They also release themselves in a pulsatile manner throughout the hour, day, or month. The circadian rhythm sets these pulsatile releases. You could consider melatonin to be something of a reset button for your body's circadian rhythm. It allows your body to recover and repair itself from wear and tear brought on throughout the day by granting you sleep. An important thing to remember about this hormone, however, is the fact that it only comes when deep states of sleep are delved into. This means that it is of the utmost importance to get lots of good, deep sleep in order to keep your endocrine system balanced.

A lot of the same things that deregulate estrogen levels also throw the entire endocrine system off of its balance. Some of these factors will be covered here:

- Inadequate sleep throws off the balance of your endocrine system as lack of sleep reduces your melatonin levels. Inadequate sleep can also lead to a number of other health complications as well. These include memory loss (both long term and short term), lack of concentration, lack of creativity, lack of problem-solving skills, moods swings (which can lead to chronic disorders such as anxiety and depression in a lot of cases), increased risk of accidents of all types, a weakened immune system, high blood pressure (especially if you sleep for 5 hours or less a night), increased risk of diabetes (blood sugar spikes when you do not get enough sleep because your body does not produce enough insulin), weight gain (neurotransmitters that tell your body when it is full are negatively impacted by sleep deprivation), low sex drive, higher risk of heart disease (inadequate sleep increases blood pressure and inflammation), and poor balance and coordination (relating to higher risk of accidents).

- Environmental pollutants such as makeup, estrogens found in water bottles, smoking, unfiltered drinking water, plastics, heavy metals, paint fumes, pesticides, and exhaust fumes. These pollutants not only affect the health of your endocrine system but also your overall health. Ozone pollution, for example, can cause congestion, chest pain, throat inflammation, cardiovascular disease, and respiratory disease. Approximately 14,000 deaths per day are attributed to water pollution. These usually occur in developing countries as a result of untreated sewage in the drinking water. Oil spills often cause rashes and skin irritation. Noise pollution is a major cause of sleep disturbance, stress, high blood pressure, and, of course, hearing loss. No matter the type of pollution a person is exposed to, adverse physical effects are bound to ensue.

- Inadequate levels of vitamin D can wildly imbalance the endocrine system. This vitamin serves as a modulator for the entire system and when you do not get enough vitamin D intakes, as many people who work indoors don't, your endocrine system can suffer.

- Emotional asymmetry is a common feature of endocrine imbalance. The endocrine system controls the flow of numerous neurotransmitters (such as GABA, dopamine, and serotonin), as well as all of your body's hormones. When this system is not working properly, any number of emotional turbulence can occur and without warning either. This can, in turn, throw the functioning of all of your body's other systems into chaos if it is not dealt with promptly.

Stress can have a number of adverse effects on your overall health. Among these is endocrine deregulation. Stress causes, among other things, a constant rise of cortisol being transmitted from the adrenals. This will continue to occur in excess until the source of the stress is tackled in a healthy way. All of this excess cortisol production is especially destructive because it consumes lots of nutrients that could otherwise be used for in the production of other hormones (such as progesterone and estrogen). This also burns through many vitamins and nutrients such as vitamin C, Zinc, the B vitamins, etc.

The quickest and easiest way to regulate your endocrine system is to eat well. This will also solve/manage many other health problems that you may have. In the case of hormone production, healthy fats are the most important things to include in your diet as cholesterol is what hormones survive off of. Avoid low-fat diets as well as unhealthy saturated fats. Instead, choose unsaturated fats and omega fatty acids. This will regulate your endocrine system as well as any supplements you will find on the market, and do so naturally too.

In regards to regulating your endocrine system, keep in mind that your body and the systems that inhabit it all have to work together in unison to keep the whole healthy. All these various parts and aspects include nutritional, genetic, environmental, physical, emotional, and mental areas of concern, among many others. You sometimes have to differentiate and specify what exactly is not working properly with your body to make progress on improving your overall health. There are, however, two main things that will improve your overall health above all other methods. A platitude that is always heard but rarely adhered to: 'eat right and exercise.'

Chapter Three: Estrogen Dominance in Men, the Disease's Effects on Men and the Fatality of the Disease

It is necessary to first confirm that male bodies do indeed produce estrogen, as well as progesterone. Estrogen dominance does not just affect women. Levels of estrogen in a man can be elevated or depressed just as they can be in a woman.

The importance of estrogen in a man's body is often severely overlooked. This hormone, among other things, regulates a man's levels of testosterone, his bone health, several brain functions, skin health, his cholesterol levels, cardiovascular functions, and his sexual function/libido.

Usually, the levels of estrogen in relation to the levels of testosterone within a man's body are finely regulated. When estrogen levels increase to an unhealthy extent, testosterone usually decreases. These two happenings can cause many different symptoms that often overlap, making it hard to distinguish what is actually happening to the body. Here are some of the symptoms of estrogen dominance in men:

- Sexual dysfunctions (decreased erectile functioning, decreased morning erections, and low libido)
- Breasts being enlarged
- Symptoms from the lower urinary tract, often as a result of benign prostatic hyperplasia (BPH)
- An increase in abdominal fat (which is also a symptom of lowered levels of estrogen)
- Feeling restless
- Reduction of muscle mass

- Type 2 diabetes
- Emotional turbulence, namely depression, and anxiety

As you can see, many of these symptoms are similar to the ones mentioned in the chapters on estrogen dominance in women and are just as harmful. Arguably the most disconcerting symptom listed here is the heightened risk of developing type 2 diabetes. This increased risk is independent of a man's testosterone levels, so it is only high estrogen levels in this case that raise this risk. In men, estrogen dominance increases the risk of developing autoimmune diseases or prostate cancer as well.

Now that we have delved into some of the symptoms of the disease in men, it may be beneficial to look at some of the most common causes of estrogen dominance to get a perspective on what to watch out for. Here are some of the most common causes for high estrogen levels in men:

- Aging
  Aromatase, an enzyme that converts testosterone into estrogen, increases as a man gets older. Interestingly enough, older men are often shown to have higher levels of estrogen than do postmenopausal women.

- Decreased muscle relative to fat
  An increase in fat, accompanied by a loss of lean muscle, is another common result of aging, as well as obesity, type 2 diabetes, and other metabolic disorders. Not only does fat often store estrogen, but it also stores aromatase, which creates even more estrogen with its conversion process. In addition, fat also stores excess estradiol. All three of these factors make excess body fat a boon to estrogen dominance.

- Testosterone therapy treatments
  It is more often than not that men who are injected with synthetic testosterone develop higher levels of estrogen shortly afterward. This is especially true in cases in which the man is given excess testosterone or is obese.

- Faulty feedback loops
  When abnormally high levels of estrogen are reached in a man's body, the brain can often be tricked into producing even less testosterone in response. The result of this mistaken response can be a systemic feedback loop which can leave a man's endocrine system in complete disarray.

While estrogen levels are almost always lower in men, having too little estrogen can harm a man just as having too much. As was the case for women, a lot of the symptoms of low estrogen levels in men are similar to those of high estrogen levels. Some of these symptoms include a lowered of sex drive/libido, an increased risk of metabolic diseases, diabetes, and cardiovascular disease, as well as decreased bone strength and an increased risk of fractures.

Both estrogen and testosterone serve specific purposes in a man's overall health. The key to the health of your endocrine system lies in the balancing of these two hormones, as well as all others. Some of the best tips for balancing out a man's endocrine system are listed below:

  o Stick to a diet of cruciferous vegetables.

These vegetables include turnip greens, bok choy, Brussel sprouts, cabbage, cauliflower, and broccoli. All of these include high doses of glucosinolates which the body transforms into bioactive compounds which also help the body increase the estrogen detoxification and decrease estrogen activity.

- o Use indole-3-carbinol (I3C) and 3,3′-diindolylmethane (DIM) as supplements.

- o The best way to supplement your cruciferous vegetable intake is with 200 mg a day of I3C as well as 100 mg a day of DIM.

- o Make sure to get sufficient amounts of vitamin B12, betaine, folate, and choline.
  These nutrients are what are called methyl donors. These help in improving a biochemical process which is called methylation, which serves as one of the most important mechanisms of estrogen metabolism and detoxification. All of these can be found in supplement form at most supermarkets, but reliable dietary sources of these nutrients include quinoa, beets, spinach, eggs, shellfish, fish, and meat.

- o Reduce weight, exercise, and increase fiber intake.

These are other ways to decrease estrogen levels in men as well as improve overall health.

If you are experiencing any of the symptoms listed above, try applying some of the remedies also mentioned here. If none of the help to alleviate your symptoms then you should consider seeing a healthcare professional about your problems.

One of the most concerning aspects of estrogen dominance and other hormonal dysfunctions is that they are potentially fatal. To understand why and how the symptoms of these dysfunctions can sometimes reach a point of fatality we must take an in-depth look at the endocrine system and its many functions.

There are also a number of other hormone-related diseases that are associated with the deregulation of your endocrine system. These include but are not limited to sexual dysfunctions, thyroid disease, growth disorders, and even diabetes.

Each gland included within the endocrine system produces and releases hormones specific to it throughout the body via the bloodstream. We will now take a look at each one of these glands:

- Adrenal glands
  These are two glands which are located around the higher end of the kidneys and release the stress hormone known as cortisol. This hormone is responsible for assessing threats and finding appropriate physiological responses to them.

- Hypothalamus
  An important part in the middle lower brain which communicates to the pituitary gland the appropriate times at which to release certain hormones.

- Ovaries
  This is the reproductive organ of a female equivalent to male testes. It releases eggs and female sex hormones, such as estrogen and progesterone.

- Islet cells located within the pancreas
  These cells in the pancreas are responsible for the release of glucagon and insulin. These hormones regulate blood sugar levels and break glycogen down into glucose for digestion in the liver respectively.

- Parathyroid
  Four very small glands located within the neck which plays a major role in the building and fostering of bone health and growth.

- Pineal gland
  A gland located around the brain's center region which is commonly linked to sleeping patterns. This is because it produces melatonin, the main hormone responsible for sleep.

- Pituitary gland
  A gland located near the brain's base, behind even the sinuses. This is commonly referred to as the 'master' gland because of the influence that it asserts over many other glands of the endocrine system, the thyroid, to name one. The main hormones that this gland releases are human growth hormones, thyroid stimulating hormones, and luteinizing hormones. Dysfunction of the pituitary gland tends to have effects on the release of a woman's breast milk, the woman's menstrual cycles, and her bone health.

- Testes
  This male sex organ is equivalent to female ovaries responsible for the production of sex hormones such as testosterone and sperm.

- Thymus
  A gland located near the upper region of the chest which builds the strength of a person's immune system early in life by producing lots of T cells to foster immune health. This gland usually shrinks in size at the onset of puberty.

- Thyroid
  A gland shaped like a butterfly found in the front of the neck which creates hormones that are responsible for regulating the body's metabolism.

Even the slightest disturbance in the functioning of one or multiple glands mentioned here can throw the entire system off of its course. This can, in turn, lead to endocrine disorder or endocrine disease. The two main culprits for the cause of endocrine disorders would have to be the following:

1. When too little or too much of a certain hormone is produced within the endocrine system. This is typically called a hormone imbalance.

2. When lesions (such as tumors or nodules) are developed on or within certain glands in the endocrine system. These lesions may or may not have any effects on hormone levels.

The endocrine system also has something of a feedback system which helps to regulate the hormonal balance within your bloodstream. If too little or too much of a specific hormone is detected within the bloodstream at any given time, this feedback system will send signals to the appropriate gland or glands to address the problem promptly. If this feedback system fails to maintain the proper amount of specific hormones in the bloodstream, however, then hormonal imbalances will occur. This will also happen when your body does not clear these hormones out of your bloodstream properly. There are many different causes of imbalances in endocrine hormone levels, some of which are included here:

- Issues involving the endocrine feedback system.

- Disease (of all kinds).

- Failure to stimulate the release of hormones from one gland to another (issues involving the hypothalamus tend to disturb the hormonal productions of the pituitary gland, for example).

- Multiple endocrine neoplasia (MEN) or congenital hypothyroidism, as well as many other genetic disorders.

- Infection (in all regions and of all sorts).

- Injury sustained by a gland within the endocrine system.

- A tumor on an endocrine gland.

- Most lesions (whether they be tumors or nodules) found in the endocrine system are benign. It is also rare that they metastasize throughout other parts of the body. These stationary and noncancerous lesions are still dangerous, however, as they can affect the hormone production of the entire system.

Now that we have looked at some of the various causes of endocrine disorders, it would be beneficial to go over what some of these disorders are and how they can affect the human body. A list of just a few of these disorders is featured below:

- Adrenal insufficiency
  Adrenal glands in this state do not produce enough of the cortisol hormones and sometimes aldosterone for the body to function properly. This can cause a wide range of symptoms, including skin changes, dehydration, upset stomach, and fatigue. One example of adrenal insufficiency would be Addison's disease, a disease which tends to cause dizziness upon standing and darkening of the skin among other things.

- *Cushing's disease*
  The overproduction of hormones by the pituitary gland often leads the overactivity of adrenal glands. Cushing's disease (or Cushing's syndrome) is a similar condition to this which often affects people, children in particular, who take higher doses of corticosteroid medications. This causes an excess of the hormone cortisol throughout the body and can be potentially fatal.

- Issues regarding growth hormones, such as gigantism (or acromegaly).

These issues usually occur when the pituitary gland produces too many growth hormones and a person's (usually a child's) body parts and bones start to grow too fast as a result. On the other hand, if growth hormones are too low, then a child can tend to stop growing in height. As with any other facet of endocrine health, the balance remains the key.

- Hyperthyroidism
This is when the thyroid produces too much of its own thyroid hormone. It often results in nervousness, sweating, increased heart rate, and weight loss. Some of these symptoms are due to increased metabolism, a result of the deregulation of the thyroid. A very common result of hyperthyroidism is an autoimmune disorder by the name of Grave's disease. This disease is most common in women over the age of 40 and its symptoms are puffy eyes, weight loss, heat sensitivity, hand tremors, and anxiety among other things.

- Hypothyroidism
This is the opposite of the previously mentioned hyperthyroidism. This is when there is an insufficiency in the amount of thyroid hormone produced. Common symptoms of this disorder include depression, dry skin, constipation, and fatigue. An underactive thyroid can cause a slowing of physical development among children. Some of the types of hypothyroidism are even diagnosable at birth.

- Hypopituitarism
This is when the pituitary gland produces little to no hormones. This is especially problematic when considering the importance of the pituitary gland

within the endocrine system. This can be caused by several different factors and or diseases and women who develop this disorder often stop having their periods.

- Multiple endocrine neoplasia 1 and 2 (MEN 1 and 2)
  These are rare genetic diseases which are often passed down through multiple generations. They are known to cause tumors and other lesions on the thyroid, adrenal, and parathyroid glands, which often lead to hormonal overproduction and endocrine imbalances.

- Polycystic ovary syndrome (PCOS)
  This disease is usually caused by the overproduction of androgens. These tend to infringe on the development of a woman's eggs and her menstrual cycle. Some of the symptoms of this disease are obesity, acne, excess hair growth (even facial hair growth), and menstrual irregularity. PCOS is also a growing cause of infertility.

- Early puberty
  When glands regulate the release of sex hormones too early in life, puberty can occur at a much younger age than usual.

Some of these disorders are self-diagnosable to an extent, but it is always better to consult a healthcare professional when it comes to endocrine disorders. If you are then found to suffer from an endocrine disorder, your doctor may then suggest that you see an endocrinologist. An endocrinologist is a doctor specifically trained in confronting issues regarding the endocrine system.

As you can tell from the symptoms mentioned above, endocrine disorders cause a wide variety of health problems which depend on the gland or glands being affected. There are common threads among different disorders as far as symptoms are concerned though, such as fatigue and weakness. These two are minor though in comparison to other symptoms brought on by these disorders.

Blood and urine tests are the most common methods among doctors of figuring out whether or not a patient suffers from an endocrine disorder. In addition, imaging tests may be administered upon confirmation of an endocrine disorder to locate any tumors or nodules that the sufferer might have.

The treatment of endocrine disorders may at times be complicated or even harmful, as when one hormone level is heightened or lowered there is a high probability of the whole system being thrown out of order. This is just one more reason to speak with a doctor about dealing with one of these disorders. Even with a healthcare professional on board, complications can easily arise at any time. Going about dealing with endocrine disorder alone only increase your chances of having to deal with unexpected adverse side effects.

When considering the multifariousness of the effects of endocrine disorders, it becomes even more unbelievable that fatality rates for these disorders aren't even higher than they already are. That is not to say that these fatality rates are especially high though. Some of the complications of endocrine disorders, such as estrogen-dependent cancers and diabetes, are obviously more problematic and lead to more deaths than other ones.

Typically endocrine disorders are somewhat easily cured and have low fatality rates, though the innumerable complications of these disorders tend to make things harder for those who live with them.

On the whole, endocrine disorders can be overcome and people can live long, healthy lives beyond their stints with these disorders. There can, however, be potentially disastrous consequences of developing these disorders though, so early intervention and careful care need to be made and taken when dealing with these disorders.

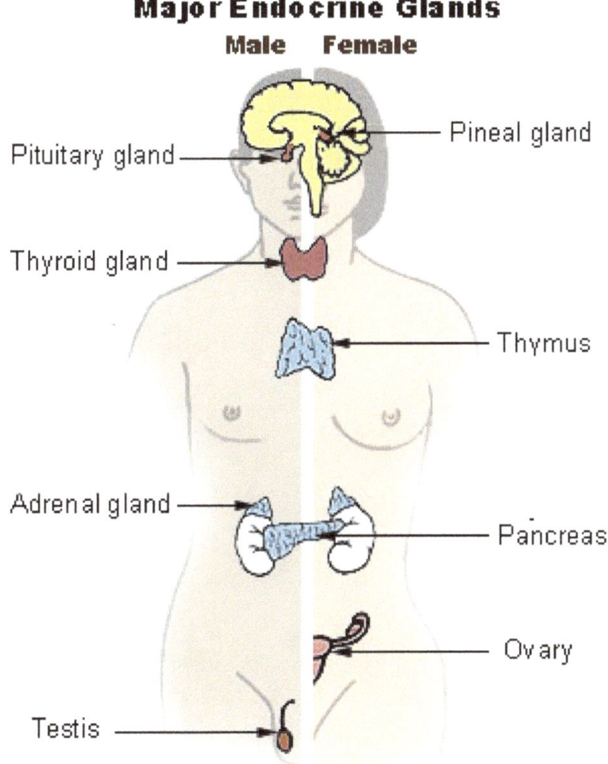

Chapter Four: Coping with Estrogen Dominance and What to Do After You Conquer It

There have been some general dieting tips previously included within this book on dealing with estrogen dominance at large, but now it should be delved into what some of the foods are which are helpful to eat to alleviate some of the more severe symptoms of this disease.

To start off, some of the best natural foods to eat if you develop breast cancer, breast lumps, and or fibroids as a result of estrogen dominance are listed below. These foods naturally balance estrogen and progesterone levels and are also helpful for liver functioning.

- Chaste tree

Chaste tree, also commonly called monk's pepper, received these names for its anti-aphrodisiac properties. Monks used to chew the leaves and berries of this plant to help them control their urges. This is because, when consumed in large quantities, this plant is shown to decrease libido. One of the best features of this plant is the fact that it contains luteinizing hormones which raise progesterone levels and therefore lower estrogen levels. This plant can alleviate constipation, headache, depression, bloating, and painful, lumpy breasts.

- Passionflower

This is a flower high in a naturally occurring flavonoid which may help to lower estradiol called chrysin. This plant is great for women with postmenopausal sleep disturbances because it lowers estradiol and has natural calming and sedative qualities.

- Raspberry leaf

This is a leaf rich in its levels of an antioxidant by the name of ellagic acid. This leaf can also alter estrogen metabolism rates, reducing the risk of development of many hormonal cancers.

- Maca

Maca root is what is known as a 'herbal adaptogen', like ginseng and or licorice. It is so titled because it adapts to your body's hormonal needs, assisting your endocrine system in regulating your body's hormones. Women who ingest maca or maca supplements are often shown to have increased in progesterone levels, and therefore decrease in estrogen levels.

- Brussel sprouts and broccoli

Broccoli helps to inhibit breast cancer stem cells, according to some research. This also prevents new tumors and nodules from formulating as it contains a compound by the name of sulforaphane.

One other nasty symptom of estrogen dominance is poor liver functioning. While estrogen usually has no trouble circulating itself throughout the body, it sometimes can become lodged within the liver in excess. This causes the liver to lose its ability to filter out any harmful estrogen metabolites, which the organ is usually able to do easily. When the liver is rendered unable to perform this task the entire endocrine system can be thrown off balance. Below we will go over some of the most helpful foods in combating liver issues surrounding estrogen.

- Milk thistle

This plant helps your liver to remove excess amounts of estrogen and can even lower levels of cholesterol.

- Artichoke

This is a plant which will help your body's production of bile. This bile will, in turn, help your liver with the elimination of excess bile.

- Dandelion leaf and root

This is a bitter plant which will further stimulate your bile production to facilitate the detoxification process in your liver. This will help not only estrogen but also progesterone byproducts consumption and their removal from the body, usually by excretion.

- Cruciferous vegetables

These include plants like broccoli, cauliflower, arugula, and kale, all of which are known to contain glucosinolates, which in turn activate phase 2 of detoxification in the liver, the filtering of estrogen metabolites from your body. These vegetables may also help you if you suffer from thyroid issues. This is because if you cook any of these then around 80% of their goitrogenic chemicals will leave them.

One of the more severe mood-altering symptoms of estrogen dominance is PMS. One of the effects of this disorder is that women who suffer from it can experience violent mood swings during their menstrual cycles. Fluid retention, as well as breast tenderness, are two additional effects of PMS. These are all caused by hormonal turbulence within the endocrine system and they can have devastating results. When both PMS and estrogen dominance are experienced simultaneously, the result can be a severely reduced quality of life which can lead to even further complications.

Some of the best foods to eat for alleviating PMS symptoms are listed below:

- Seeds

Beyond all of the foods mentioned above, seeds are virtually the only additional foods helpful in combating PMS symptoms. Symptoms of estrogen dominance can also be reduced very much by seed cycling. Seeds can also provide many important vitamins and nutrients in the production of hormones, providing a boon to the entire endocrine system. Among these are zinc and vitamin E. A proper amount of these would be around one to two tablespoons with each soup, salad, smoothie, etc. that you make. It also remains important to learn what your body requires and what is most beneficial for you to eat by trial and error. The types of seeds you should eat vary with which hormones you are trying to boost, and which ones you are trying to reduce.

If you are trying to boost your estrogen levels, these would be the best seeds for you to eat:

  - Pumpkin and flax seeds
    Boosting estrogen is more important to do throughout days 1-14 of the menstrual cycle, so eating these seeds during that time period is important.

On the other hand, the best seeds for you to eat if you are trying to boost your progesterone levels are:

o Sunflower and sesame seeds
Boosting progesterone throughout days 15-28 of the menstrual cycle is more important, so that time period is when these should be eaten.

Now that we have gone over some of the best ways to cope with symptoms of estrogen dominance as well as other hormone-related disorders, it would be helpful to look at some of the best ways to manage a balanced endocrine system beyond just balancing our estrogen levels. This should give you some useful information regarding staying healthy in the future.

Here are some of the most important steps in maintaining healthy and balanced hormone levels:

- Make sure to get enough protein at every meal.
Getting enough protein in your diet is important because dietary protein contains essential amino acids which help to maintain skin, bone, and muscle health. Protein also has influence over the release of hormones which control food intake and appetite. This 'hunger hormone' goes by the name of ghrelin, and it stimulates other hormones which control food intakes, such as PYY and GLP-1.

- Exercise regularly.
Two of the most beneficial things that regular exercise can do for your hormonal health are reducing insulin levels and increasing insulin sensitivity. Insulin has several different functions. For one, it enables cells to absorb sugar and amino acids from the bloodstream, which are then used for maintaining energy and muscle mass. Too much insulin, however, can have harmful consequences such as inflammation, heart disease, diabetes, and even cancer.

Some of the greatest types of exercise for increasing insulin sensitivity are endurance exercise, strength training, and aerobic exercise. In addition, physical exercise increases hormones which maintain muscles such as testosterone, IGF-1, growth hormones, and DHEA.

- Avoid refined carbs and sugar.

Avoiding or limiting consumption of these foods may help to optimize hormone balance and fend off diabetes, obesity, and other diseases. High fructose levels may actually increase insulin levels and lead to increased resistance to insulin.

Following a low to moderate carb diet based primarily on whole foods may lead to a decrease in insulin levels and in insulin resistance. This is especially true for obese or overweight people.

- Manage stress properly.

Stress can wreak just as much havoc on your endocrine system as a poor diet can. The two main hormones the stress produces are cortisol and adrenaline, also known as an epinephrine. Cortisol helps your body cope with long-term stress and is therefore called the 'stress hormone'. Adrenaline, on the other hand, provides your body with the short-term storage of energy in desperate situations and is therefore called the 'fight or flight' hormone.

Chronic stress can lead to a number of health complications, including the long-term elevation of cortisol levels, which can, in turn, lead to excess calorie intake and therefore weight gain. While long-term elevation of adrenaline levels is less common, their short-term effects are just as if not more so severe. Excess adrenaline can cause anxiety, rapid heart rate, and high blood pressure.

Stress reducing techniques such as yoga, meditation, massages, and listening to relaxing music are the best ways to reduce cortisol and adrenaline levels. It is always advisable to devote 10-15 minutes a day to these techniques, even if it is hard to make such a time.

- Only consume healthy fats.

Avoiding unnatural and unhealthy fats may help reduce appetite and insulin resistance. Medium chain triglycerides (or MCTs) are healthy fats which are absorbed by the liver and used for energy production. They are also known to reduce insulin resistance. MCTs can usually be found in palm and coconut oils. Monounsaturated and dairy fats are also known to increase insulin sensitivity. These can usually be found in olive oils and nuts. Consuming healthy fats at meals also release hormones which keep you feeling full and satisfied, like CCK, PYY, and GLP-1.

- Avoid under and overeating.

Neglecting to eat in a balanced way can result in hormonal imbalances which can cause weight problems, among other things. Overeating, especially carbs and sugars can dramatically increase your insulin levels. On the other hand, under eating can result in increased cortisol production, resulting in weight gain and other hormonal imbalances.

- Drink green tea.

Green tea boasts a wide variety of health benefits. Among these is caffeine which boosts metabolism, and an antioxidant known as epigallocatechin gallate (or EGCG).

The consumption of green tea both increases insulin sensitivity and lowers insulin levels.

• Eat fatty fish as often as possible.
Fatty fish is the best naturally occurring source of omega-3 fatty acids, which are shown to have beneficial anti-inflammatory effects. In addition, fatty fish also has beneficial effects on hormonal health, including reducing the levels of cortisol and adrenaline in the body.

Those who suffer from gestational diabetes, obesity, and polycystic ovary syndrome also receive benefits from eating omega 3 fatty acids. These include the increase of insulin resistance.

The most popular species of fish with high-fat content which provide omega-3 fatty acids are mackerel, herring, sardines, and salmon.

• Make sure to get consistent, high-quality sleep.
A lack of restorative sleep will negate any of the positive effects of trying any of the techniques mentioned above. Lots of hormonal imbalances, including those regarding growth hormone, ghrelin, leptin, cortisol, and insulin can easily be caused by a lack of deep sleep.

When adequate amounts of sleep are not met, insulin sensitivity often decreases, leptin levels decrease, and ghrelin levels increase. Appetite also starts to skyrocket and weight is often gained.

Your brain requires lots of uninterrupted sleep throughout all five stages of brainwave activity involved in sleep. This is of special importance for the production of growth hormone. For the best hormone balance, a minimum of seven hours of sleep a night is necessary.

- Avoid sugary beverages.

Sugar is typically unhealthy in any given form. The liquid sugars appear to be the unhealthiest of any kinds. Drinks that have excess amounts of liquid sugars have been shown to increase insulin resistance. Drinking sugary beverages also leads to excess weight gain because of the fact that these beverages do not send out the same signals which communicate fullness as other foods. Avoiding these beverages is one of the easiest and most beneficial steps that you can take in maintaining hormonal balance.

- Keep a high amount of fiber in your diet.

Not only does a high amount of fiber increase insulin sensitivity, but it also produces higher levels of the hormones which make you feel full, often leading to substantial weight loss. Soluble fiber is the type that has the most profound effects on eating and appetite, however, insoluble fiber plays an important role in these respects as well.

In overweight and obese people, eating a type of soluble fiber by the name of oligofructose has been shown to increase levels of PYY, while the consumption of cellulose, an insoluble fiber, has been shown to increase levels of GLP-1.

- Include lots of eggs in your diet.

Overall, eggs are one of the most nutrient-packed foods that you can get your hands on. As far as hormone production is concerned, eggs are shown to decrease levels of ghrelin and insulin, as well as increase levels of PYY.

Those who eat eggs for breakfast usually report feeling fuller and eat fewer calories throughout the day. Whole eggs tend to boast more health benefits than egg whites do though. Eating whole eggs have been shown to increase insulin sensitivity and even improve overall heart health.

Eggs are typically eaten only at breakfast. They can, however, be enjoyed with any meal and at any time of the day.

Conclusion

Thank you for making it through to the end of Estrogen Dominance: Natural Remedies and Healthy Living. Let's hope that the information provided here proves to be of some help to you. Among all of the topics discussed here, there should be at least one thing which helps you in some way.

The next step in maintaining your endocrine health would be to apply these principles to your everyday life, namely the dieting tips. If all of these are adhered to persistently, some results should come out of all of this. If none of these tips benefit you or do not do enough for you, then consider searching for other resources on this topic. There are plenty of them out there on the market.

 On the whole, endocrine disorders can be overcome and people can live long, healthy lives beyond their stints with these disorders. There can, however, be potentially disastrous consequences of developing these disorders though, so early intervention and careful care need to be made and taken when dealing with these disorders.

If at first, you see no results in practicing the main principles laid out in this book, then stay persistent in them and you may find that some benefits do occur.

Description

If you are experiencing symptoms of an endocrine disorder of any kind then this is the book for you. The main disorder covered in this book, however, is estrogen dominance. In this book, we will go over some answers for some of the following questions: what is estrogen dominance? What are some of the best ways to combat the disease and heal from it naturally? What are some of the effects of high and low estrogen? Is this disease fatal? Are women the only sex to suffer from estrogen dominance? How do you cope with it? What do you do after you conquer it?

Estrogen dominance is a complex issue for a person to face. It is generally defined as the state in which the amount of estrogen is greater than that of progesterone in the body. This is typically caused by a decrease in a person's level of progesterone without a complementary decrease in his or her level of estrogen. There is, however, no set guideline on the amount of excess estrogen that constitutes estrogen dominance. It is determined by the amount of estrogen in relation to other sex hormones.

Where there exists an excess or deficiency of any specific hormone throughout the body's endocrine system, overall imbalances start to occur and health problems start to rear their heads. Among other situations, this can occur when there is too much estrogen in a person's system and not enough progesterone to counteract it all.

Not only does estrogen dominance plague women, but males are also susceptible to the disorder. The importance of estrogen in a man's body is often severely overlooked. This hormone, among other things, regulates a man's levels of testosterone, his bone health, several brain functions, skin health, his cholesterol levels, cardiovascular functions, and his sexual function/libido.

Usually, the levels of estrogen in relation to the levels of testosterone within a man's body are finely regulated. When estrogen levels increase to an unhealthy extent, testosterone usually decreases. These two events can cause many different symptoms that often overlap, making it hard to distinguish what is actually happening to the body.

As you can already tell, estrogen dominance and other endocrine disorders are incredibly complex problems which take lots of studies to get a grasp of. In downloading this book you will/have gained a valuable resource in understanding more about these issues.